Preface

Welcome to "Home Workouts: Effective Exercises for Fitness and Fat Loss"! In a world where time is a precious commodity and the demands of our daily lives seem to constantly increase, finding the motivation and opportunity to prioritize our health and well-being can be a challenge. However, with the right knowledge and tools, achieving your fitness goals doesn't have to be an insurmountable task.

In this eBook, I aim to provide you with a comprehensive guide to home workouts that will help you not only improve your fitness levels but also shed unwanted fat. Whether you are a beginner looking to kick-start your fitness journey or someone with prior experience seeking new workout routines, this book is designed to be your ultimate resource.

My name is Arinze Cyril, and I have been a fitness enthusiast and personal trainer for over a decade. I have witnessed first-hand the transformative power of exercise, and I am passionate about sharing my knowledge and expertise to help others achieve their fitness aspirations. Throughout the pages of this eBook, I have distilled years of experience and research into a practical, easy-to-follow guide that can be implemented within the confines of your own home.

Why home workouts, you may ask? Well, the answer is simple. Not everyone has access to a gym or the luxury of time to commute back and forth. However, with the right guidance, your home can become your fitness sanctuary—a place where you can challenge yourself, build strength, and burn fat effectively. By eliminating the obstacles of location and time, this eBook empowers you to take control of your fitness journey and make tangible progress, all within the comfort of your own space.
Inside these pages, you will find a variety of exercises and workout routines tailored to different fitness levels, from beginners to advanced. You will learn how to perform each

exercise correctly, ensuring optimal results while minimizing the risk of injury. I will also provide insights into the science behind effective workouts and how they contribute to fat loss and overall fitness.

In addition to exercise routines, I will also touch on other important aspects of fitness, including nutrition tips and lifestyle recommendations that will support your goals. After all, achieving fitness and fat loss requires a holistic approach that goes beyond just physical activity.

Remember, the key to success lies in consistency and commitment. The journey to a healthier, fitter version of yourself begins with the decision to take action. By incorporating the exercises and principles outlined in this eBook into your daily routine, you will be on your way to transforming your body and improving your overall well-being.

I am thrilled to embark on this journey with you, and I hope that this eBook serves as a valuable resource to help you achieve your fitness goals. Remember to listen to your body, stay motivated, and celebrate your progress along the way. Let's embark on this transformative adventure together, one workout at a time!

Stay fit, stay focused, and let's get started!

Arinze Cyril

Table of contents

A. Importance of warm-up and its benefits B. Dynamic warm-up exercises to prepare the body C. Stretching routines to enhance flexibility and prevent injuries

VI. Cardiovascular Exercises for Fat Loss

A. Explanation of cardio's role in burning fat B. Different types of cardio exercises for home workouts C. Structuring effective fat-burning cardio sessions.

VII. Strength Training for Building Muscle and Burning Fat

A. Benefits of strength training for fat loss and overall fitness B. Introduction to bodyweight exercises and resistance training C.

Designing strength training workouts for different muscle groups

VIII. HIIT (High-Intensity Interval Training) Workouts

A. Understanding the principles and benefits of

HIIT B. Sample HIIT workouts for maximizing calorie burn C. Tips for incorporating HIIT into home workout routines

IX. Creating Balanced Workout Programs

A. Developing workout schedules and routines B. Balancing cardio, strength training, and recovery days C. Progression and adaptation for long-term results

X. Nutrition Tips for Fitness and Fat Loss

A. Importance of proper nutrition in conjunction with exercise B. Guidelines for healthy eating and portion control C. Fueling the body for optimal performance and fat loss

XI. Staying Motivated and Overcoming Challenges

A. Strategies for maintaining motivation in home workouts B. Dealing with plateaus and adjusting workout intensity C. Building a support system and celebrating achievements

XII. Conclusion

A. Recap of key points and takeaways B. Encouragement for readers to start their home workout journey C. Final thoughts on the benefits of home workouts for fitness and fat loss.

Introduction

Welcome to "Home Workouts: Effective Exercises for Fitness and Fat Loss," an eBook designed to help you achieve your fitness goals from the comfort of your own home. In this comprehensive guide, we will explore the importance of home workouts, the benefits of exercising for fitness and fat loss, and provide you with practical exercises and routines to transform your body and improve your overall well-being.

Chapter II

begins by differentiating between fitness and fat loss goals and explaining the crucial role that exercise plays in achieving both. We will also delve into setting realistic expectations, ensuring that you have a clear understanding of what you can achieve through home workouts. Setting up an ideal workout space is essential

Chapter III

guides you through the process. From assessing available space and equipment options to creating a safe and functional environment, you will discover how to optimize your home for effective workouts. Additionally, we offer valuable tips for staying motivated in a home workout setting, ensuring that you remain dedicated to your fitness journey.

Chapter IV

focuses on essential home workout equipment. We provide an overview of basic equipment that can enhance your workouts and offer recommendations for budget-friendly options. Furthermore, we explore alternatives for exercises that require no equipment, allowing you to adapt your routine to your resources. Prior to diving into the exercises,

Chapter V
emphasizes the importance of warm-up and stretching. You will learn about the benefits of a proper warm-up and discover dynamic warm-up exercises to prepare your body for the workout ahead. Additionally, we provide stretching routines to enhance flexibility and prevent injuries.

Chapter VI

explores cardiovascular exercises specifically targeted for fat loss. We explain the role of cardio in burning fat and introduce different types of cardio exercises that can be easily performed at home. Moreover, you will learn how to structure effective fat-burning cardio sessions for optimal results. Building muscle and burning fat go hand in hand, and in

Chapter VII

we delve into the benefits of strength training. From bodyweight exercises to resistance training, you will discover how to incorporate these exercises into your routine for maximum impact. We also guide you in designing strength training workouts that target different muscle groups.

HIIT (High-Intensity Interval Training) is the focus of **Chapter VIII**, where we explore its principles and benefits. You will find sample HIIT workouts designed to maximize calorie burn and receive valuable tips for seamlessly integrating HIIT into your home workout routines.

Chapter IX

takes a holistic approach to fitness by guiding you in creating balanced workout programs. We explore the importance of developing schedules and routines that incorporate cardio, strength training, and recovery days. Additionally, we provide insights into progression and adaptation to ensure long-term success.

In Chapter X, we shift our focus to nutrition, recognizing its vital

role in conjunction with exercise. You will gain an understanding of healthy eating guidelines and portion control, enabling you to fuel your body optimally for performance and fat loss. Maintaining motivation and overcoming challenges are crucial to sustaining a home workout routine, and

Chapter XI

offers strategies to help you stay on track. We address common plateaus and provide tips for adjusting workout intensity. Furthermore, we highlight the significance of building a support system and celebrating achievements along the way.

Finally, in Chapter XII,

we recap the key points and takeaways from this eBook. We offer encouragement to embark on your home workout journey, knowing that a healthier, fitter version of yourself awaits. We conclude by reiterating the benefits of home workouts for fitness and fat loss and leave you with final thoughts to inspire and motivate you on your path to success.

Get ready to transform your body, enhance your fitness, and achieve your fat loss goals with "Home Workouts: Effective Exercises for Fitness and Fat Loss." Let's embark on this journey together and unlock your full potential.

Chapter 2

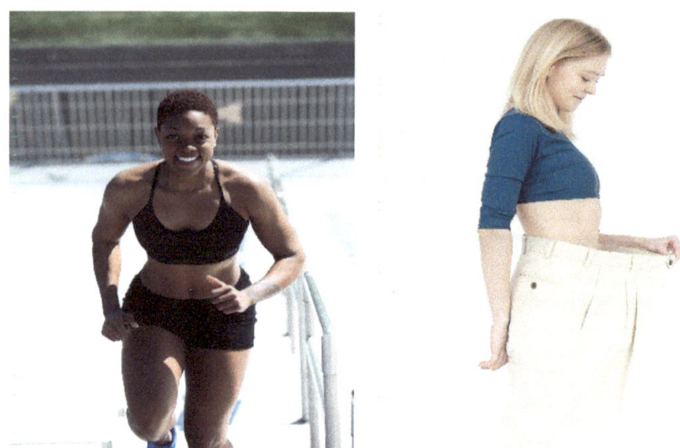

Understanding Fitness and fat loss

1. Differentiating between Fitness and Fat Loss Goals:

When it comes to improving our health and wellbeing, it's essential to understand the distinction between fitness fat loss goals. While they are related, they involve different aspects of our overall physical condition.

Fitness goals encompass improving cardiovascular endurance, muscular strength, flexibility, and overall physical performance. These goals focus on enhancing our body's ability to perform various activities and maintain a healthy lifestyle. Examples of fitness goals may include running a certain distance without stopping, increasing the number of push-ups you can do, or improving your flexibility to touch your toes.

On the other hand, fat loss goals primarily revolve around reducing body fat percentage and achieving a leaner physique. This entails losing excess weight and inches around specific areas, such as the waist or thighs. Fat loss goals are often associated with aesthetic improvements and improving body composition.

While fitness and fat loss goals may overlap in some areas, it's crucial to identify which aspect you prioritize more. Understanding your goals will help you tailor your workouts and make better decisions regarding exercise selection, intensity, and nutrition.

2. The Role of Exercise in Achieving Fitness and Fat Loss Goals:

Exercise plays a pivotal role in achieving both fitness and fat loss goals. It not only helps to burn calories but also contributes to building strength, endurance, and overall physical fitness. Here are some key points to consider:

A.Caloric Expenditure: Exercise helps create a caloric deficit, which is crucial for fat loss. By engaging in physical activities that elevate your heart rate, such as aerobic exercises, you burn calories, leading to weight loss and a reduction in body fat percentage.

B.Muscle Development: Resistance training exercises, such as weightlifting or bodyweight exercises, are instrumental in building and toning muscles. While aerobic exercise burns calories during the activity, strength training helps increase your muscle mass, which can boost your metabolism and help you burn more calories even at rest.

C.Cardiovascular Health: Regular aerobic exercise improves your cardiovascular endurance, strengthens your heart, and enhances the efficiency of your cardiovascular system. This is crucial for overall fitness, as it allows you to perform daily tasks with less fatigue and increases your capacity for more intense workouts.

D.Functional Movement: Exercise helps improve your coordination, balance, and flexibility, enabling you to move more efficiently and with reduced risk of injury. Functional movements, such as squats, lunges, and core exercises, contribute to both fitness and fat loss goals by enhancing your overall physical performance and stability.

3. Setting Realistic Expectations

While exercise is essential for achieving fitness and fat loss goals, it's important to set realistic expectations to avoid frustration or discouragement. Here are some key considerations:

A. Differences: Everyone's body is unique, and individuals will respond differently to exercise and dietary changes. Factors such as genetics, age, current fitness level, and overall health can impact your progress. Therefore, it's crucial to focus on your own journey and not compare yourself to others.

B.Sustainable Progress: Rapid weight loss or significant muscle gain in a short period is often unrealistic and may not be healthy. It's essential to adopt a sustainable approach to your fitness and fat loss journey. Aim for gradual progress, such as losing 1-2 pounds per week or increasing your strength and endurance gradually over time.

C) Non-Scale Victories: Remember that progress extends beyond the numbers on the scale. Celebrate non-scale victories such as increased energy levels, improved mood, better sleep quality, or fitting into clothes more comfortably. These achievements are just as significant and should be acknowledged.

d) Lifestyle Changes: Achieving long-term success requires adopting healthy lifestyle habits beyond exercise alone. Focus on incorporating a balanced diet, adequate sleep, stress management.

Chapter 3

Setting up Your Home Workout space

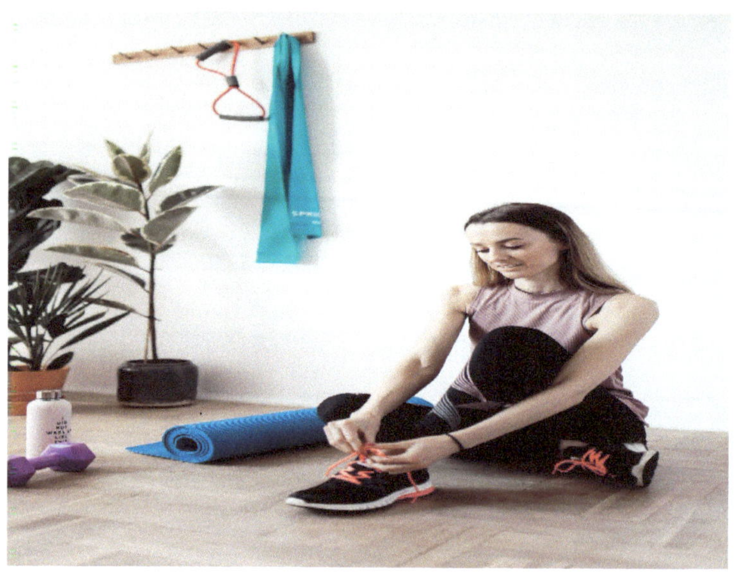

1.Assessing Available Space and Equipment Options

When it comes to setting up your home workout space, it's important to assess the available space and choose the right equipment options that suit your needs and fitness goals. Here are some considerations to keep in mind:

A.Space Assessment: Start by evaluating the amount of space you have in your home. Measure the dimensions of the room or area where you plan to set up your workout space. Consider the ceiling height as well, especially if you plan to incorporate exercises that require overhead movements.

B.Equipment Selection: Based on the space available, select the appropriate workout equipment that aligns with your fitness goals. Some popular options include:

Cardio Machines: If you enjoy cardiovascular exercises, consider equipment such as treadmills, stationary bikes, or elliptical trainers. These machines provide a great way to burn calories and improve your cardiovascular fitness.

Resistance Training: For strength training, you can opt for dumbbells, resistance bands, kettle bells, or a home gym system. Choose equipment that suits your current fitness level and allows you to perform a variety of exercises.

Bodyweight Exercises: Don't underestimate the power of bodyweight exercises. They require minimal space and can be highly effective. Include equipment like a yoga mat, stability ball, or pullup bar for added versatility.

Remember, the key is to choose equipment that fits your available space and aligns with your workout preferences. Quality over quantity is essential, so invest in equipment that will withstand regular use and help you achieve your fitness goals.

2. Creating a Safe and Functional Workout Environment

Once you've selected your equipment and determined the space, it's crucial to create a safe and functional workout environment within your home. Here are some tips to ensure your setup is optimal:

A.Flooring: Choose a suitable flooring option that provides stability, cushioning, and grip. Options like rubber mats or interlocking foam tiles work well to protect your joints and prevent equipment from sliding.

B.Ventilation and Lighting: Ensure the area is well-ventilated with proper airflow to keep you comfortable during workouts. Adequate lighting is also essential for safety and visibility. Natural light is ideal, but if that's not possible, invest in good quality lighting fixtures.

C.Storage and Organization: Keep your workout space tidy and organized. Use storage solutions like shelves, hooks, or bins to store your equipment neatly. This will not only create a clutter-free environment but also help you locate and access your equipment easily.

D.Safety Measures: Consider safety measures such as securing heavy equipment to prevent tipping, ensuring electrical outlets are located away from water sources, and placing a first aid kit nearby in case of emergencies. If you have children or pets at home, create a designated workout space that is out of their reach.

3. Tips for Staying Motivated in a Home Workout Setting

Maintaining motivation is key to achieving success with your home workouts. Here are some tips to help you stay motivated and make the most of your home workout space:

A.Set Clear Goals: Define your fitness goals and write them down. Whether you aim to lose weight, build muscle, or improve overall fitness, having specific goals will provide you with a sense of purpose and direction.

B.Establish a Routine: Create a consistent workout routine and schedule it into your daily or weekly calendar. Treating your home workouts with the same level of commitment as you would a gym session will help you stay on track.

C.Find Accountability: Share your fitness journey with a friend, family member, or join an online fitness community. Having someone to hold you accountable and provide support can significantly increase your motivation.

D.Vary Your Workouts: Avoid monotony by incorporating a variety of exercises into your routine.

Chapter 4

Essential Home Workout Equipment

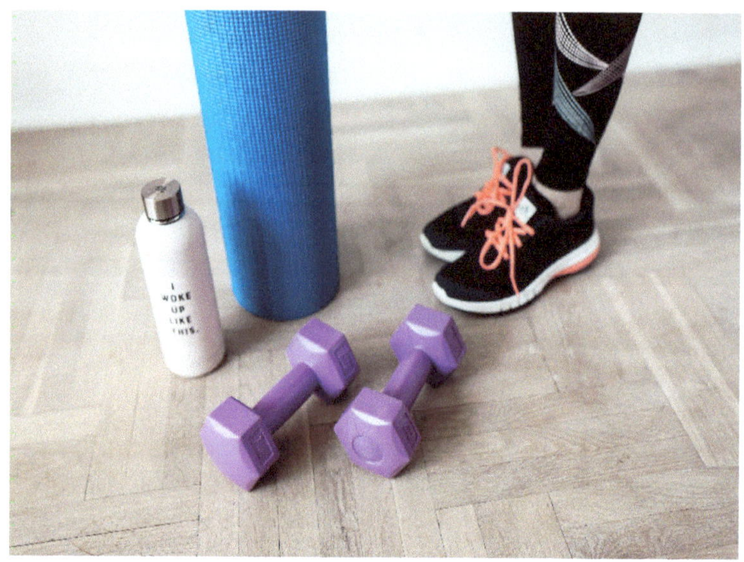

In this chapter, we will explore the basic equipment that can enhance the effectiveness of your home workouts. Whether you're aiming for overall fitness or targeting fat loss, having the right tools at your disposal can make a significant difference in achieving your goals. We'll discuss budget-friendly options and alternatives for exercises that don't require any equipment.

1. Overview of Basic Equipment for Effective Workouts

When setting up your home gym, it's essential to invest in a few key pieces of equipment to enhance your workout routine. Here are three essential items that can provide a solid foundation for effective home workouts:

A.Resistance Bands: Resistance bands are versatile and affordable exercise tools that come in various levels of resistance. They can target different muscle groups and provide resistance throughout the entire range of motion. With resistance bands, you can perform exercises such as bicep curls, squats, lateral walks, and more. They are lightweight, portable, and suitable for individuals of all fitness levels.

B.Dumbbells: Dumbbells are excellent for strength training and building muscle. They come in different weights, allowing you to choose the appropriate level of resistance for each exercise. Dumbbells can be used for various exercises, including shoulder presses, lunges, chest presses, and rows. Investing in a set of adjustable dumbbells can save space and money, as you can increase or decrease the weight by simply adjusting the plates.

C.Stability Ball: A stability ball, also known as an exercise or Swiss ball, is a versatile piece of equipment that improves core stability and balance. It can be used for a wide range of exercises, such as crunches, planks, push-ups, and lower body exercises like squats and lunges. Additionally, sitting on a stability ball instead of a chair can engage your core muscles and improve posture while working or watching TV.

2. Recommendations for Budget-Friendly Options

If you're on a tight budget, there are affordable alternatives to expensive exercise equipment. Here are some budget-friendly options that can still provide an effective workout:

A.Bodyweight Exercises: Bodyweight exercises require no equipment and utilize the resistance of your own body to build strength and improve fitness. Exercises like push-ups, squats, lunges, planks, and burpees can be performed anywhere, making them a cost-effective option for home workouts.

B.Water Bottles or Milk Jugs: Water bottles or milk jugs filled with water or sand can serve as makeshift weights. You can hold them in your hands for exercises like bicep curls, overhead presses, or use them as weights for squats and lunges. They are readily available and can be adjusted in weight by adding or removing water or sand.

C.Resistance Bands: As mentioned earlier, resistance bands are an affordable alternative to traditional weightlifting equipment. They provide resistance similar to weights and can be used for various exercises targeting different muscle groups. They are often sold in sets with varying levels of resistance, allowing you to gradually increase the challenge as you progress.

3. Alternatives for Exercises without Equipment

If you prefer not to invest in any equipment or are looking for alternatives when you can't access your usual workout gear, don't worry. There are plenty of exercises that can be performed without any equipment. Here are a few examples:

A. Exercises: Activities like jogging, jumping jacks, high knees, mountain climbers, and burpees can elevate your heart rate and provide a great cardio workout without any equipment.

B.Bodyweight Exercises: As mentioned earlier, bodyweight exercises are highly effective for strength training. Include exercises like push-ups, squats, lunges, planks, and glute bridges in your routine to target different muscle groups.

Chapter 5

Warm-up and stretching

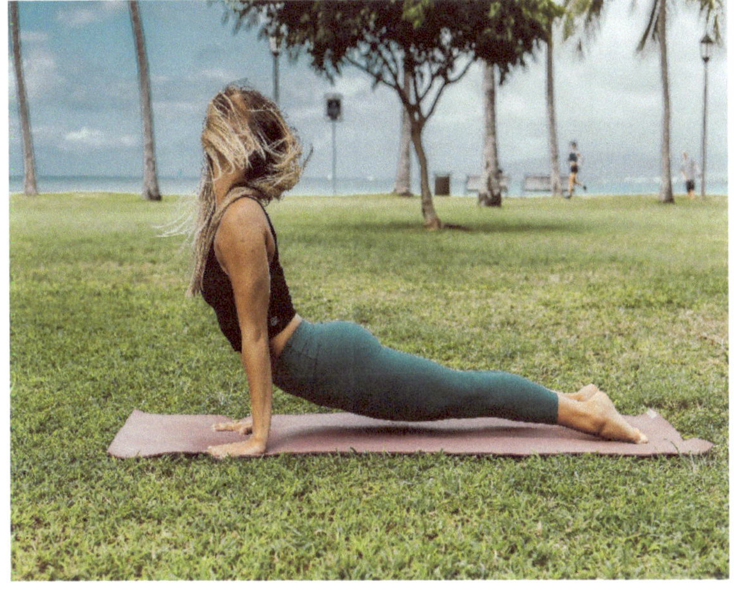

Introduction: In order to maximize the effectiveness of your home workouts and ensure your safety, it's crucial to pay attention to the warm-up and stretching routines. Warm-up exercises and stretching play a vital role in preparing your body for exercise, enhancing flexibility, and reducing the risk of injuries. In this chapter, we will explore the importance of warmup, discuss its benefits, introduce dynamic warmup exercises, and provide stretching routines that will help you achieve your fitness goals while staying safe.

1. Importance of Warm-up and Its Benefits:

 Before diving into the main workout, it's important to warm up your body. The warm-up phase gradually increases your heart rate, boosts blood flow to the muscles, and raises your body temperature. This prepares your body for the upcoming physical activity by activating the neuromuscular system, enhancing joint mobility, and improving muscular function. Here are some key benefits of incorporating a proper warm-up into your exercise routine:

A.Injury Prevention: A thorough warm-up increases the flexibility and elasticity of your muscles, tendons, and ligaments. This reduces the risk of strains, sprains, and other injuries during your workout.

B.Improved Performance: By increasing your heart rate and blood flow, a warm-up enhances oxygen delivery to your muscles. This helps improve muscle performance, speed, agility, and overall exercise capacity.

C.Mental Preparation: Warm-up exercises provide an opportunity to mentally prepare for your workout. It helps you shift your focus from daily activities to the task at hand, improving concentration and boosting motivation.

2. Dynamic Warm-up Exercises to Prepare the Body:

Dynamic warm-up exercises involve moving your body through a range of motions that mimic the movements you'll be performing during your main workout. These exercises help to activate and engage the muscles, lubricate the joints, and increase the heart rate. Here are some dynamic warm-up exercises you can incorporate into your routine:

a. **Arm Circles:** Stand with your feet shoulder width apart. Extend your arms straight out to the sides and make small circles with your arms. Gradually increase the size of the circles, and then reverse the direction.

b. High Knees: Stand tall and start jogging in place, lifting your knees as high as possible while keeping your torso upright. Aim for quick, controlled movements.

c. **Lunges with a Twist:** Take a step forward with your right leg into a lunge position. As you lower your body, rotate your torso to the right. Return to the starting position and repeat on the other side.

d. **Jumping Jacks:** Begin with your feet together and your arms by your sides. Jump and spread your feet wider than hip-width apart while simultaneously raising your arms overhead. Jump back to the starting position and repeat.

Remember to perform each exercise for about 1015 repetitions or for a duration of 30 seconds to 1 minute. Gradually increase the intensity as you progress.

3. Stretching Routines to Enhance Flexibility and Prevent Injuries:

Stretching after your warm-up and workout helps to improve flexibility, reduce muscle soreness, and prevent muscle imbalances. Here are a few stretching routines to incorporate into your home workout routine:

a. **Standing Hamstring Stretch:** Stand tall with one leg extended straight in front of you on an elevated surface. Keep your back straight and gently lean forward from your hips until you feel a stretch in the back of your extended leg. Hold for 20-30 seconds, then switch legs.

b. **Quadriceps Stretch:** Stand tall and grab your right ankle, pulling it toward your glutes until you feel a stretch in the front of your thigh. Keep your knees together and your torso upright. Hold for 20-30 seconds, then switch legs.

c. **Chest Stretch:** Certainly! Here's how you can perform a chest stretch:

I.   Stand tall with your feet shoulder-width apart.

II. Extend your arms straight out to the sides, parallel to the floor, with your palms facing forward.

III. Take a deep breath in and exhale slowly as you bring your shoulder blades together.

IV. As you bring your shoulder blades together, gently squeeze your shoulder blades down and back.

V. You should feel a stretch across your chest and the front of your shoulders.

VI. Hold the stretch for 20-30 seconds while maintaining a relaxed breathing pattern.

VII. Release the stretch and repeat as needed.

Tips:

I. Make sure to keep your back straight and your core engaged during the stretch.

II. Avoid shrugging your shoulders or straining your neck.

III.   If you feel any pain or discomfort, ease off the stretch and adjust your position.

The chest stretch helps counteract the forward posture often caused by prolonged sitting or desk work. By stretching the chest muscles, you can improve your posture and alleviate tension in the upper body. Incorporating this stretch into your routine after your warm-up and workout can contribute to overall flexibility and prevent imbalances.

Chapter 6

Cardiovascular Exercises for Fat Loss

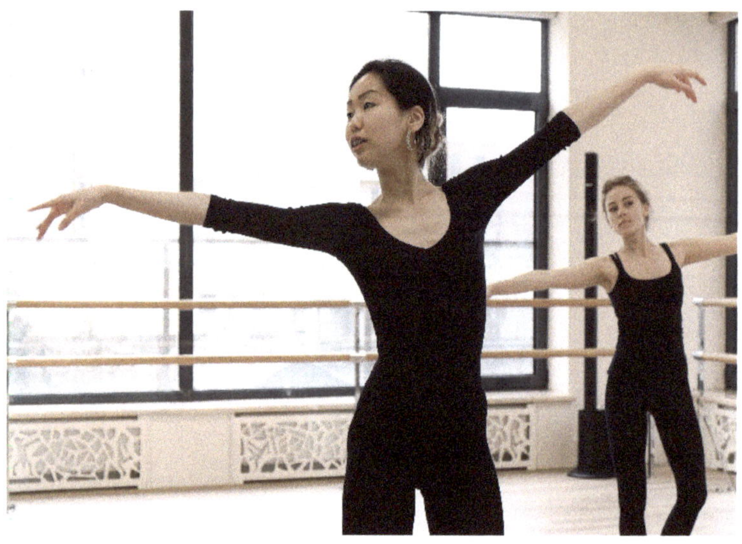

Introduction: In the quest for achieving optimal fitness and shedding excess body fat, cardio exercises play a vital role. Cardiovascular exercises, also known as cardio, are a fantastic way to elevate your heart rate, increase your metabolism, and burn calories effectively. In this chapter, we will explore the significance of cardio in fat loss, various types of cardio exercises suitable for home workouts, and how to structure effective fat-burning cardio sessions to help you achieve your fitness goals.

1. Explanation of Cardio's Role in Burning Fat:

Cardio exercises are highly effective for burning fat due to their ability to elevate your heart rate and increase energy expenditure. When you engage in cardio, your body requires additional energy to sustain the increased level of activity, which primarily comes from stored fat cells. As a result, regular cardio workouts create a calorie deficit, leading to fat loss over time. Additionally, cardio exercises help improve cardiovascular health, boost endurance, and enhance overall wellbeing.

2. Different Types of Cardio Exercises for Home Workouts:

A. High-Intensity Interval Training (HIIT): HIIT workouts involve alternating short bursts of intense exercise with periods of active recovery. They are an excellent option for burning fat in a short amount of time. HIIT exercises like jumping jacks, burpees, mountain climbers, and high knees can be performed effectively at home, requiring minimal or no equipment.

B. **Bodyweight Cardio Circuits:** Bodyweight cardio circuits combine strength training exercises with cardio movements. They are ideal for improving muscular endurance while burning calories. Examples of bodyweight cardio exercises include squat jumps, jumping lunges, mountain climbers, and plank jacks.

C. **Dance Fitness:** Dancing is a fun and engaging way to incorporate cardio into your home workouts. You can follow dance workout videos or freestyle to your favorite tunes. Dancing not only elevates your heart rate but also enhances coordination and boosts mood.

D. **Skipping Rope:** Skipping rope is a simple yet highly effective cardio exercise that can be performed indoors. It engages multiple muscle groups, improves cardiovascular fitness, and burns a significant amount of calories. Start with a comfortable pace and gradually increase the intensity and duration as you progress.

E. **Cardio Machines:** If you have access to cardio machines like a treadmill, stationary bike, or elliptical trainer, they can be excellent options for home workouts. These machines provide a controlled and customizable environment to perform cardio exercises, allowing you to adjust the intensity, duration, and resistance according to your fitness level.

3. Structuring Effective Fat-Burning Cardio Sessions:

To structure an effective fat-burning cardio session, consider the following tips:

A.Warm-up: Begin with a 5-10 minute warm-up to prepare your body for exercise. This can include light jogging, marching in place, or dynamic stretching to loosen up the muscles.

B.Choose the Right Intensity: The intensity of your cardio workout is crucial for fat loss. Aim for a moderate to high intensity that challenges your cardiovascular system. This can be achieved through intervals of high-intensity exercise alternated with periods of active recovery or steady-state cardio at a challenging pace.

C.Vary Workouts: To prevent boredom and ensure continuous progress, vary your cardio exercises regularly. Mix different types of cardio workouts mentioned earlier or try new exercises to keep your body and mind engaged.

C.Incorporate Resistance Training: Combining cardio with resistance training exercises can maximize fat loss and help maintain lean muscle mass. Include bodyweight exercises, resistance bands, or light dumbbells in your cardio sessions to add a strength-training element.

D.Progress Gradually: As your fitness level improves, gradually increase the duration, intensity, or frequency of your cardio workouts. This progressive overload helps challenge your body and ensures continuous fat loss.

Chapter 7

Strength Training for Building Muscle and Burning Fat

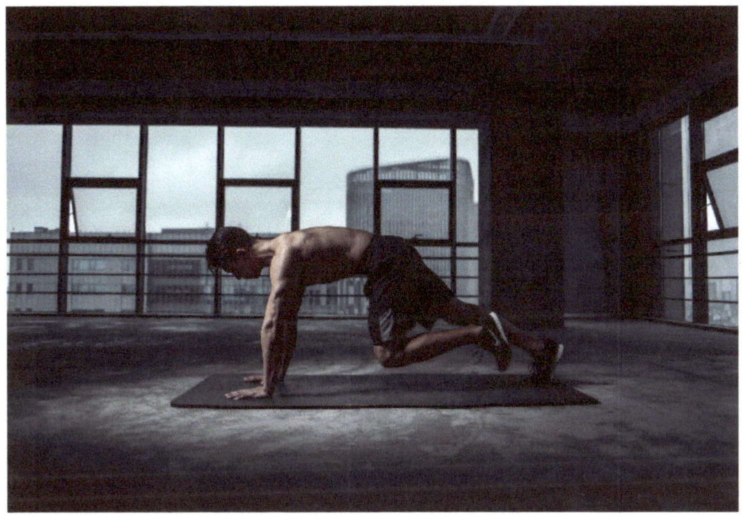

Introduction: In this chapter, we will delve into the world of strength training and its incredible benefits for both muscle building and fat loss. We will explore the advantages of strength training, introduce you to bodyweight exercises and resistance training, and guide you in designing effective strength training workouts for different muscle groups. Get ready to sculpt your body and achieve your fitness goals!

1. Benefits of Strength Training for Fat Loss and Overall Fitness:

Strength training is a powerful tool for transforming your body composition and improving overall fitness. Here are some key benefits of incorporating strength training into your workout routine:

A.Increased Muscle Mass: Strength training stimulates muscle growth, leading to an increase in lean muscle mass. More muscle mass boosts your metabolism, helping you burn more calories throughout the day, even at rest.

B.Enhanced Fat Burning: Strength training promotes the after burn effect, also known as excess post-exercise oxygen consumption (EPOC). This means that after a strength training session, your body continues to burn calories at an elevated rate for several hours, aiding in fat loss.

C. Improved Metabolic Health: Regular strength training improves insulin sensitivity, which helps regulate blood sugar levels and can reduce the risk of type 2 diabetes. It also promotes healthy cholesterol levels and lowers blood pressure.

d. Increased Strength and Functional Fitness: Strength training enhances your overall strength, making everyday activities easier. It improves bone density, joint stability, and muscular endurance, reducing the risk of injuries and enhancing overall functional fitness.

2. Introduction to Bodyweight Exercises and Resistance Training:

Strength training can be achieved through various modalities, including bodyweight exercises and resistance training. Let's take a closer look at each of them:

A.Bodyweight Exercises: These exercises utilize your body weight as resistance, making them convenient and suitable for home workouts.

Examples include push-ups, squats, lunges, planks, and burpees.

Bodyweight exercises help build muscle, increase strength, and improve flexibility.

B.Resistance Training: This form of strength training involves using external resistance, such as dumbbells, resistance bands, or weight machines.

Resistance training allows for progressive overload, where you gradually increase the resistance over time to continuously challenge your muscles and stimulate growth.

3. Designing Strength Training Workouts for Different Muscle Groups:

To effectively target and develop different muscle groups, it's important to design well-rounded strength training workouts. Here are few step guide to help you get started:

A.Set Clear Goals: Determine your specific fitness goals, whether it's building muscle, burning fat, or both. This will guide your exercise selection and intensity.

B.Choose Compound Exercises: Incorporate compound exercises that engage multiple muscle groups simultaneously. Examples include squats, deadlifts, bench presses, and pull-ups. These exercises maximize efficiency and stimulate overall muscle growth.

C.Focus on Individual Muscle Groups: Devote specific workouts or days to target different muscle groups. This approach ensures balanced development and allows for proper recovery. For example, dedicate one day to training your legs and glutes, another day for upper body exercises, and so on.

D.Incorporate Progression: Gradually increase the intensity of your workouts over time. This can be achieved by adding more resistance, increasing the number of repetitions or sets, or decreasing the rest periods between exercises.

E.Allow for Recovery: Adequate rest and recovery are crucial for muscle growth. Ensure you have rest days between strength training sessions to allow your muscles to repair and rebuild.

F.Track Your Progress: Keep a workout journal or use fitness apps to track your exercises, weights, and repetitions. This will help you monitor your progress, identify areas for improvement, and stay motivated.

Conclusion: Strength training is a fantastic way to build muscle.

Chapter 8

HIIT (High-Intensity Interval Training) Workouts

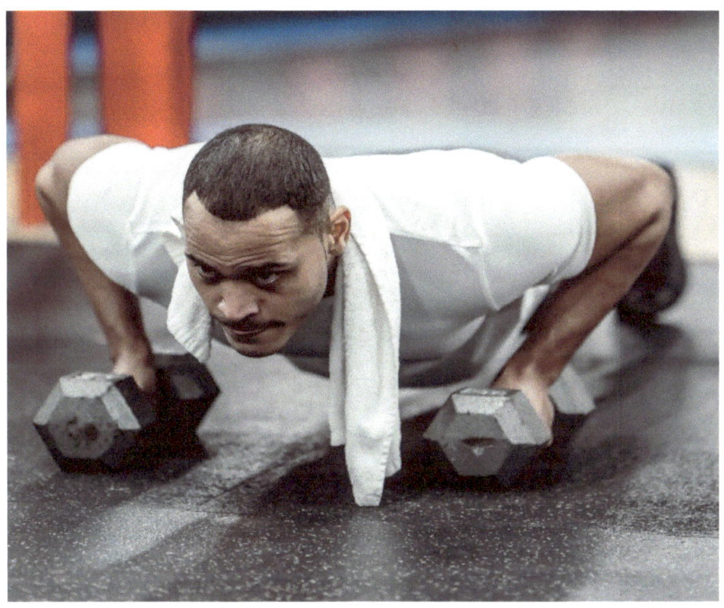

Introduction: this chapter, we will delve into the world of High-Intensity Interval Training (HIIT) workouts. HIIT has gained immense popularity in recent years due to its effectiveness in burning calories, improving cardiovascular fitness, and enhancing overall health. We will explore the principles and benefits of HIIT, provide sample workouts for maximizing calorie burn, and offer valuable tips for incorporating HIIT into your home workout routines. Get ready to push your limits and achieve remarkable results with HIIT!

Section 1: Understanding the Principles and Benefits of HIIT

1.1 The Basics of HIIT:

I. What is HIIT and how does it differ from traditional cardio workouts.

II. The concept of alternating high-intensity exercises with short rest periods.

III. The science behind the effectiveness of HIIT in burning calories and fat.

IV. The metabolic and cardiovascular benefits of HIIT.

1.2. Key Principles of HIIT:

I.   Intensity: Pushing yourself to your maximum effort during the high intensity intervals.

II.   Interval Duration: Determining the optimal length of work and rest intervals.

III.   Variation: Incorporating a mix of exercises to target different muscle groups.

IV.   Progression: Gradually increasing the difficulty of HIIT workouts for continuous improvement.

V.   Safety Considerations: Tips for avoiding injuries and listening to your body's signals.

1.3. Benefits of HIIT:

I. Efficient Time Utilization: Achieving maximum results in minimal time.

II.   Calorie Burn and Fat Loss: The impact of HIIT on metabolism and weight management.

II.   Improved Cardiovascular Fitness: Strengthening the heart and enhancing endurance.

III.   Muscle Toning and Strength: Building lean muscle mass and boosting overall strength.

IV.   Enhanced Metabolic Rate: The long-lasting calorie burn effect post workout.

V.   Adaptability and Accessibility: HIIT can be tailored to various fitness levels and performed anywhere.

Section 2: Sample HIIT Workouts for Maximizing Calorie Burn

2.1. Full-Body HIIT Circuit:

I. A circuit-style workout targeting multiple muscle groups.

II.   Exercises such as burpees, mountain climbers, squat jumps, and plank variations.

III.   A 20-minute high-intensity routine with 30 seconds of work and 15 seconds of rest.

2.2 Tabata-style HIIT Workout:

I. The Tabata protocol: 20 seconds of intense exercise followed by 10 seconds of rest.

II. Exercises like kettle bell swings, box jumps, push-ups, and bicycle crunches.

III. A 15-minute workout incorporating eight rounds of Tabata intervals.

2.3 Cardio HIIT Blast:

I. An intense cardio-focused HIIT workout to elevate heart rate and burn calories.

II. Exercises such as high knees, jumping jacks, skaters, and lateral shuffles.

III. A 25-minute routine with 40 seconds of work and 20 seconds of rest.

Section 3: Tips for Incorporating HIIT into Home Workout Routines

3.1 Establishing a Routine:

I. Finding the best time to incorporate HIIT into your daily schedule.

II. Setting realistic goals and expectations for your home HIIT workouts.

III. Creating a dedicated workout space within your home.

3.2 Equipment and Modifications:

I. Equipment options for home HIIT workouts: bodyweight exercises, resistance bands, dumbbells, etc.

II. Modifying exercises to suit your fitness level and available equipment.

III. Safety precautions for performing HIIT at home.

3.3 Progression and Variation:

I. Increasing the intensity and duration of HIIT workouts over time.

II. Incorporating different exercises and workout formats to keep things challenging.

Chapter 9

Creating Balanced Workout Programs

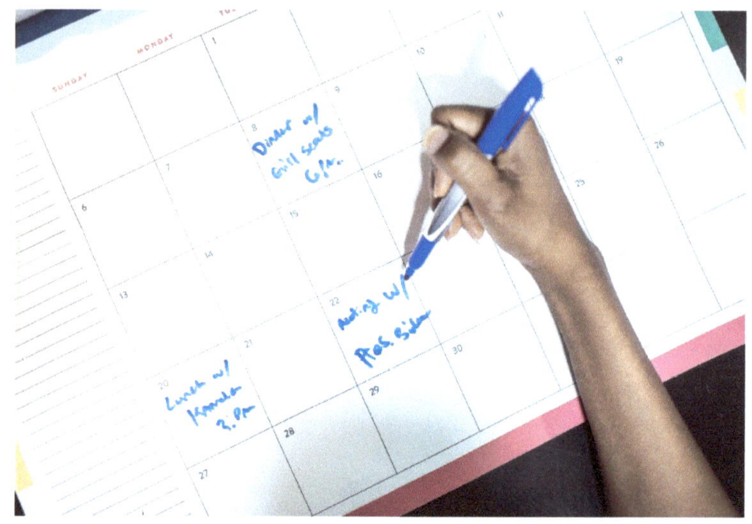

Introduction: In the previous chapters, we discussed various exercises and techniques for home workouts that are effective for fitness and fat loss. However, simply performing exercises randomly won't yield the best results. To maximize your progress and ensure long-term success, it's important to create balanced workout programs. In this chapter, we will delve into the key aspects of developing workout schedules and routines, balancing cardio, strength training, and recovery days, and understanding progression and adaptation for long-term results.

1. Developing Workout Schedules and Routines:

One of the first steps in creating a balanced workout program is to establish a schedule and routine. Consistency is key to achieving your fitness goals. Determine how many days per week you can commit to working out, considering your other commitments and responsibilities. Aim for a minimum of three to four days of exercise per week to see significant improvements. Once you have decided on the frequency, assign specific days for your workouts. For example, you might choose Monday, Wednesday, Friday, and Sunday as your workout days. Having a set schedule will help you stay on track and make exercise a regular part of your routine.

2. Balancing Cardio, Strength Training, and Recovery Days:

A well-rounded workout program includes a balance of cardio, strength training, and recovery days. Cardio exercises, such as running, cycling, or jumping jacks, help improve cardiovascular endurance and burn calories.

Strength training exercises, on the other hand, build lean muscle mass and increase overall strength. Lastly, recovery days are crucial for allowing your body to rest and repair itself.

To strike the right balance, aim for a combination of cardio and strength training exercises on alternate days. For example, you could perform cardio workouts on Monday, Wednesday, and Friday, and dedicate Tuesday, Thursday, and Saturday to strength training. This approach ensures that you work on different aspects of fitness while allowing your muscles to recover adequately. As for recovery days, consider incorporating active recovery activities like yoga or gentle stretching to improve flexibility and reduce muscle soreness.

3. Progression and Adaptation for Long-Term Results:

To continue making progress and avoid plateaus, it's essential to incorporate progression and adaptation into your workout program. Your body adapts to exercise over time, so it's necessary to challenge yourself consistently. Here are some strategies for progression:

A.Gradually increase intensity: As your fitness improves, gradually increase the intensity of your workouts. For cardio exercises, this can involve increasing the duration or speed of your sessions. In strength training, you can increase the weight, number of sets, or repetitions. This progressive overload stimulates further muscle growth and cardiovascular improvements.

B.Vary exercises and techniques: Continually challenge your body by introducing new exercises and techniques into your routine. This prevents boredom and ensures that different muscle groups are targeted. For example, if you usually perform squats, try incorporating lunges or Bulgarian split squats to engage your leg muscles in a different way.

C.Monitor and track progress: Keep a record of your workouts, noting the exercises performed, weights used, and the number of repetitions completed. This allows you to track your progress over time and make adjustments as needed. It also provides a sense of accomplishment and motivation.

D.Periodize your training: Periodization involves dividing your training into specific phases, each with a different focus. For example, you could have a strength-building phase, followed by a muscle endurance phase. Periodization helps prevent overtraining and promotes continuous improvement by targeting different fitness components.

Conclusion: Creating balanced workout programs is crucial for achieving long-term results. By developing workout schedules and routines, balancing cardio, strength training, and recovery days, and incorporating progression and adaptation, you can optimize your fitness journey. Remember, consistency, variety, and gradual progression are very vital for success.

Chapter 10
Nutrition Tips for Fitness and Fat Loss

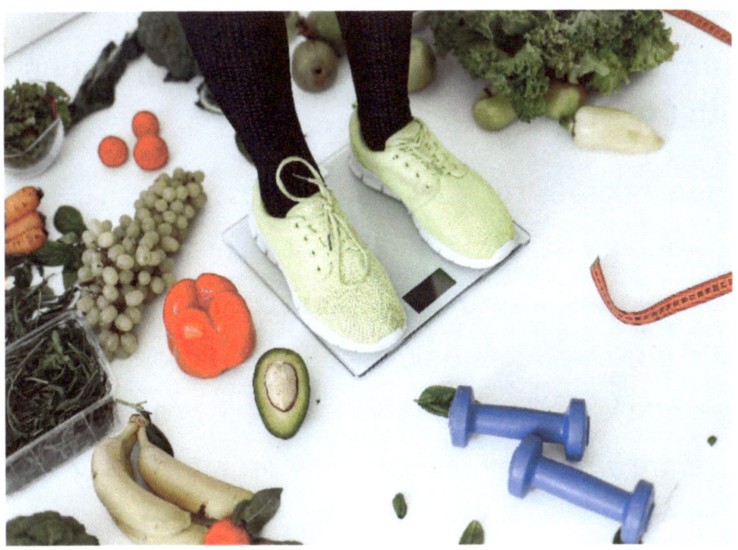

Introduction: In the previous chapters, we discussed various effective exercises for fitness and fat loss that can be performed in the comfort of your own home. However, exercise alone is not enough to achieve your desired results. Proper nutrition plays a crucial role in conjunction with exercise when it comes to optimizing performance, promoting fat loss, and maintaining overall health. In this chapter, we will delve into the importance of proper nutrition, provide guidelines for healthy eating and portion control, and explore how to fuel your body for optimal performance and fat loss.

1. Importance of Proper Nutrition in Conjunction with Exercise:

When it comes to fitness and fat loss, exercise and nutrition go hand in hand. While exercise helps to burn calories, improve cardiovascular health, and build muscle, nutrition provides the necessary fuel, nutrients, and support for these processes. Here are a few key reasons why proper nutrition is crucial:

A.Energy Balance: To achieve fat loss, it's essential to create a calorie deficit, where you consume fewer calories than you burn. Proper nutrition helps you strike the right balance between providing enough energy for exercise and ensuring a calorie deficit for fat loss.

B.Muscle Recovery and Growth: Exercise creates micro-tears in your muscles, and nutrition provides the building blocks necessary for repair and growth. Adequate protein intake is particularly important to support muscle recovery and development.

C.Nutrient Absorption and Overall Health: Proper nutrition ensures that your body receives the necessary vitamins, minerals, and micronutrients for optimal function. A well-balanced diet can support your immune system, enhance recovery, and reduce the risk of chronic diseases.

2. Guidelines for Healthy Eating and Portion Control:

To optimize your nutrition for fitness and fat loss, it's important to establish healthy eating habits and practice portion control. Here are some guidelines to follow:

A.Eat Whole, Nutrient-Dense Foods: Focus on consuming whole foods that are rich in nutrients, such as fruits, vegetables, lean proteins, whole grains, and healthy fats. These foods provide essential vitamins, minerals, fiber, and antioxidants while keeping you satisfied.

B.Practice Portion Control: Be mindful of your portion sizes to avoid overeating. Use smaller plates, measure your food, and listen to your body's hunger and satiety cues. It's also helpful to avoid distractions while eating, such as watching TV or using electronic devices.

C.Balance Macronutrients: Include a balance of macronutrients in your meals. Aim for a combination of lean proteins, complex carbohydrates, and healthy fats. Proteins help with muscle repair and satiety, carbohydrates provide energy, and fats support hormone production and nutrient absorption.

D.Stay Hydrated: Drink an adequate amount of water throughout the day to support digestion, metabolism, and overall health. Hydration is especially important during exercise to maintain performance and prevent dehydration.

3. Fueling the Body for Optimal Performance and Fat Loss: To maximize your performance during workouts and promote fat loss, consider the following tips:

A.Pre-Workout Nutrition: Consume a balanced meal or snack that includes carbohydrates and protein about 1-2 hours before exercising. This will provide you with sustained energy and prevent muscle breakdown during workouts.

B.Post-Workout Nutrition: After exercising, prioritize consuming a combination of protein and carbohydrates within 30 minutes to promote muscle recovery and glycogen replenishment. This could be a protein shake, a balanced meal, or a snack like Greek yogurt with fruits.

C.Healthy Snacking: Opt for nutrient-dense snacks such as fruits, vegetables with hummus, nuts, or Greek yogurt. These options provide satiety, energy, and essential nutrients without sabotaging your fat loss goals.

Chapter 11

Staying Motivated and Overcoming Challenges

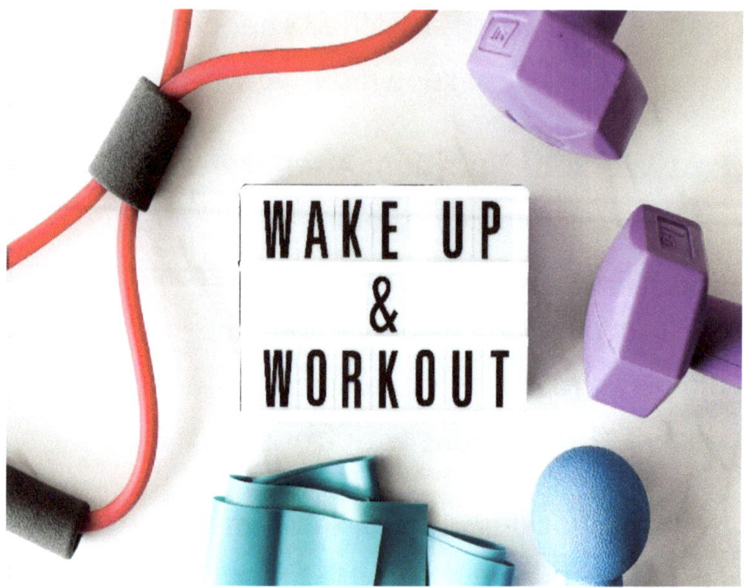

Introduction: Congratulations on reaching Chapter 11 of "Home Workouts: Effective Exercises for Fitness and Fat Loss." By this point, you have learned numerous exercises and routines to help you achieve your fitness goals. However, maintaining motivation and overcoming challenges is an ongoing process. In this chapter, we will explore strategies for staying motivated in your home workouts, dealing with plateaus, adjusting workout intensity, building a support system, and celebrating your achievements. Let's dive in!

1. Strategies for Maintaining Motivation in Home Workouts: Staying motivated can be challenging, especially when the allure of the couch or distractions at home can easily sidetrack you. Here are some strategies to help you stay motivated:

A.Set Clear Goals: Define your fitness goals and write them down. Make them specific, measurable, achievable, relevant, and time-bound (SMART). Regularly remind yourself of these goals to maintain focus and motivation.

B.Create a Routine: Establish a consistent workout schedule that aligns with your daily routine. By incorporating workouts as a regular part of your day, they become ingrained habits, making it easier to stay motivated.

C.Mix It Up: Avoid monotony by varying your workouts. Incorporate different exercises, try new workout routines, or explore fitness classes online. Variety keeps things fresh and exciting, preventing boredom and enhancing motivation.

D.Track Progress: Keep a workout journal or use fitness apps to track your progress. Seeing improvements, such as increased repetitions, heavier weights, or improved endurance, can be incredibly motivating and reinforce your efforts.

E.Find Inspiration: Follow fitness influencers, join online communities, or participate in virtual fitness challenges. Surrounding yourself with likeminded individuals who share similar goals can provide motivation, inspiration, and support.

2. Dealing with Plateaus and Adjusting Workout Intensity: Plateaus are common in any fitness journey, and they can be frustrating. However, with the right approach, you can overcome them and continue progressing:

A.Assess Your Routine: Evaluate your current workout routine to identify any patterns or areas that may be causing the plateau. Look for opportunities to challenge your body differently, such as adding new exercises, increasing intensity, or trying different training techniques.

B.Adjust Intensity: Gradually increase the intensity of your workouts by adding resistance, increasing repetitions or sets, shortening rest periods, or incorporating high-intensity interval training (HIIT) into your routine. These adjustments will challenge your body and break through plateaus.

C.Cross-Training: Incorporate cross-training into your routine by engaging in activities such as swimming, cycling, or yoga. These activities work different muscle groups and provide a refreshing change to your regular workouts.

D.Rest and Recovery: Sometimes, plateaus occur due to overtraining or inadequate recovery. Ensure you're getting enough rest between workouts and prioritize quality sleep. Allow your body time to recover and rebuild, which can help break through plateaus.

3. Building a Support System and Celebrating Achievements:

Having a support system and celebrating your achievements are crucial for staying motivated and overcoming challenges:

A.Find an Accountability Partner: Partner up with a friend, family member, or workout buddy who shares similar fitness goals. Having someone to exercise with or hold you accountable can boost motivation and make the journey more enjoyable.

B.Join Online Communities: Participate in fitness forums, social media groups, or online communities where you can connect with individuals pursuing similar fitness goals. Share your progress, seek advice, and celebrate milestones together.

C.Celebrate Milestones: Recognize and celebrate your achievements along the way. Whether it's reaching a weight loss goal, increasing your workout duration, or mastering a challenging exercise, acknowledge your progress and reward yourself.

Chapter 12

Conclusion

Congratulations on reaching the final chapter of "Home Workouts: Effective Exercises for Fitness and Fat Loss"! Throughout this eBook, we have explored a variety of exercises and strategies to help you achieve your fitness goals from the comfort of your own home. Now, let's recap the key points and takeaways from our journey and discover the lasting benefits of incorporating home workouts into your routine.

1. Recap of Key Points and Takeaways:

In our exploration of home workouts, we have covered a wide range of exercises targeting different muscle groups and fitness objectives. From bodyweight exercises like push-ups and squats to incorporating resistance bands or dumbbells, you have learned that there are numerous options available to challenge your body and stimulate muscle growth. We have emphasized the importance of proper form and technique to prevent injury and maximize results.

Additionally, we discussed the significance of progressive overload, gradually increasing the difficulty of your workouts over time to keep pushing your limits.

Furthermore, we explored the significance of cardiovascular exercises and their role in burning calories and improving cardiovascular health. We also touched upon the benefits of incorporating high-intensity interval training (HIIT) into your routine for increased fat loss and improved endurance. Lastly, we emphasized the significance of a well-rounded approach to fitness, incorporating strength training, cardiovascular exercises, flexibility training, and rest and recovery into your workout routine.

2. Encouragement to Start Your Home Workout Journey:

Now that you have gained a comprehensive understanding of home workouts and their potential, it's time to take the leap and embark on your fitness journey. It's normal to feel a mix of excitement and trepidation as you begin something new, but remember that every journey starts with a single step. The key is to take that first step and commit yourself to the process.

You might encounter obstacles along the way, such as lack of motivation, time constraints, or the temptation to give up when progress seems slow. However, remind yourself of your goals and the reasons why you started this journey in the first place. Remember that consistency and patience are vital. Celebrate small victories and use them as fuel to keep pushing forward. Surround yourself with a supportive community or enlist a workout buddy to keep you accountable and motivated. With dedication and perseverance, you can achieve remarkable results.

3. Final Thoughts on the Benefits of Home Workouts for Fitness and Fat Loss:

Home workouts offer a multitude of benefits for individuals seeking to improve their fitness and achieve fat loss goals. By exercising at home, you eliminate the constraints of time and location, making it easier to fit workouts into your schedule. The convenience of home workouts allows you to save valuable time that would have otherwise been spent commuting to and from a gym.

Moreover, home workouts provide a comfortable and private environment, eliminating self-consciousness and allowing you to focus solely on your goals without distractions. You have the freedom to tailor your workouts to your specific needs, preferences, and fitness level. Whether you're a beginner or an experienced fitness enthusiast, home workouts can be adapted to challenge you appropriately.

By consistently engaging in home workouts, you will experience numerous physical and mental benefits. Regular exercise has been shown to improve cardiovascular health, increase muscle strength and endurance, enhance flexibility, boost metabolism, and promote fat loss. It also releases endorphins, the "feel-good" hormones, which can alleviate stress, anxiety, and depression while improving your overall mood and well-being.

In conclusion, home workouts provide a practical and effective means of achieving fitness and fat loss goals. By following the exercises and principles outlined in this eBook, you can embark on a fulfilling fitness journey that will lead you to improved health, increased confidence, and a stronger, fitter version of yourself.

Remember, the power to transform your body and your life lies within you